Fighting
with
Faith

JOSHUA SISCO

ISBN 978-1-68517-293-0 (paperback)
ISBN 978-1-68517-294-7 (digital)

Christian Faith Publishing
832 Park Avenue
Meadville, PA 16335
www.christianfaithpublishing.com

Printed in the United States of America

CONTENTS

INTRODUCTION

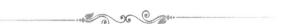

I shall begin by acknowledging that this is a book that the Lord has steered me to write. Please note that I am not a reverend, a priest, or a pastor; I am not a Christian theologian; I am not a psychologist; I am not a brilliant philosopher; I am not a medical doctor, nor am I even a famous author. Sorry if I seem to fall short of being "qualified." But God didn't think so. Who thought little David would go up against the giant Goliath and actually prevail?

Of course, that was merely the first step of David's journey with faith and finding favor with God, which ultimately led to the Davidic kingdom and many other victories for the little bullied nation of Jews. With that said, get your sling ready, my friends, and gather your stones. We are going to fight this giant beast, cancer, together.

Who am I to speak on such a matter? I am simply a Christian layman who has personally gone through two major brain surgeries (involving stage 4 cancer), who along with some experience and valuable knowledge, advice, and faith in God, knows how to string about a group of words. Upon this book's conclusion, I believe you will see that I indeed had much to offer you on the subject of cancer and faith.

Just know that what I have to offer you on both subjects is indeed more personal than professional, a point of view that I've personally found lacking in the published world with regard to this specific topic.

An unforgettable day in June of 2017 would permanently alter the rest of my life. What began with a texted photo of my face (which unbeknownst to me was drooping on the left side) led to a quick car ride to the hospital. That led to a six-hour-long emergency craniotomy, which evolved into an incredibly short five-day hospital stay wherein at some point I was told I had stage 4 brain cancer, glioblastoma.

I had never before heard the term *glioblastoma*, but I certainly knew what cancer was. It is something terrible that happens to other people, typically to people you hardly know and some whom you used to know. I will cover my own story in a bit more detail later on in this book.

Prior to that dreary morning, I lived what I would call a fairly normal American life. I had a wife and two kids. I was physically active and in extremely good shape for a thirty-five-year-old male. I ate fairly healthy and worked out five days a week. I'm here to tell you, brothers and sisters, sometimes an apple a day does not keep the oncologist away.

I wish to take a brief opportunity before you partake in this journey with me to explain my intentions to you. I want to clearly state this much: The fact that you and I both have cancer does not certify me as someone who should or even does relate to you holistically, and I would never claim to know what you're going through on a personal level.

I am, however, quite sure there are some underlying similarities in our battle against this beast of burden. However, as my audience, know that I do not presume to completely understand your own unique challenges with this fight as all cancer journeys are unique in their own regards—as are all humans. Yet we are all children of God, and that is something we should agree on.

Furthermore, this is not a book I ever believed I would or even desired to write. I prefer to write fictional stories as I still have the imagination of a child, and some might argue the demeanor as well.

Then God started hinting at me to write this. It started with a simple statement from my mother who suggested I should write a book about my story with cancer. I brushed it off. I prefer to keep my personal affairs to myself. That's just how I operate.

Then there were friends who claimed I had somehow inspired them, then there was a counselor, and what capped it off was my priest during a confession who surmised with a solution to fix the personal conundrum I had been facing with respect to writing this book.

At the time I was wrapping up my second book in a fictional series that I intend to publish publicly someday but for personal reasons am forced to hold off on doing so. Currently my oldest son, family, and friends are waiting to read it in a self-published format as a follow-up to the first book they've already read.

The priest could see that what the Lord was calling me to do appeared to be weighing heavily on me. Very bluntly and without much personal thought, he commanded me to finish the book I was writing and then begin working on this book. My so-called personal dilemma that had been burdening my already battle-worn brain seemed to have such a simple remedy when it came from the Holy Spirit. You see, I had been carrying around this great sense of guilt over wanting to finish my book before writing what the Lord wanted me to write. That guilt led to inactivity. For a while I hadn't been writing anything as my guilt impeded my motivation to do either.

Until that confession, I had been praying adamantly to the Lord to give me a sign as to whether or not I should write this book. "Ask, and it will be given to you; seek and you will find; knock and the door will open" (Matthew 7:7). Truth be told, I think I was hoping God would tell me to write whatever I wanted. However, I have surrendered myself to the will of God (a powerful life transformation that we will discuss in further detail later on), and He reminded me of that surrender through both the Holy Spirit and my priest that day in the confessional booth. He also reminded me that He doesn't call us to our vocations in order to strike us with misery. He wants us to fulfill our purpose using what He has given us to offer on His behalf.

I left the church that day full of relief and conviction knowing exactly what I needed to do. I finished that second book free from guilt and then began my journey into this book, knowing it was not my will but the Lord's will. I can tell you that the Lord's will is the greatest tour guide you will ever have on earth.

It took me many years to realize that my will might be more comparable to a rafting guide who shows up on the riverbank at nine in the morning reeking of booze with bloodshot eyes hollering, "Let's hit them rapids, boys"—the sort of guide whom you'd be afraid to climb into the raft with. And for so much of my life, I was fixated on being my own guide. I thought I knew what was best for me. In retrospect, that notion is preposterous.

My truest intention here is that you come away from reading this book having garnered some insight into your battle with cancer (or perhaps for someone you know) that will serve to prepare, uplift, and even begin your healing process through God's grace.

A cancer diagnosis does not have to be a death sentence. God is not punishing you. It's easy for some people to fall into the "blame God" trap. On a human level, it is even understandable. My first piece of advice to you is do not turn negative against the Lord. Nothing good comes from being negative about *anything* when you have cancer.

Second, please do not treat your diagnosis as a death sentence, even if your doctors do. Maybe that's a bit conspicuous to hear coming from someone who does not even know you, but I believe it is important for you to hear nonetheless.

Truly, the devil has no power over you; but when you let go of hope, you're letting go of your soul, and the body cannot sustain without the soul. Write that down.

Praise be to God, our Lord and Savior Who deserves all the credit for this book coming to fruition. I only pray that I can do it justice.

PART 1

Begin with Prayer and Understanding

CHAPTER 1

Who Do You Say That I Am?

This is a question that Jesus asked His disciples. If Jesus asked me that question today, my answer would be to smile and say, "Really, Lord? You know that I know that You are the Christ, the only begotten Son of God." If you know Jesus Christ the way I have come to know Him, this would be your answer as well.

I was debating on whether or not to even write this chapter of the book, but undoubtedly I knew that if I were to write about this, it would have to occur right here—in the beginning.

I wanted to assume that if you were to purchase this book or simply pick this book up and begin to read, you would already have a foundation of faith, but now I think perhaps this was a naive assumption on my part. Your cancer may very well be the beginning of your journey toward Christ as I've come to discover this is not uncommon.

In light of this personal conclusion, I shall begin with a brief definition of faith. It is pertinent for you to have a basic understanding of this concept in order for you to acquire anything of value from the pages that follow.

Faith is believing for sure. You cannot truly have Christian faith if you do not believe Jesus is the Son of God. But belief is simply the foundation upon which the much broader structure of what faith *really* is rests on.

I'm sure you have heard the word *strength* in one of its connotative forms associated with faith. Does this mean that if your faith is stronger, you believe in God more than one whose faith is not as strong? Perhaps, but I do not believe that is always the case.

I think it is entirely possible for two people to believe in God equally but for one of them to have stronger faith. Allow me to clarify.

I have always believed in God, for as long as I can remember. I am talking from a small child until this very day in my late thirties. But my faith wasn't always strong.

I spent most of my life attempting to be my own tour guide, and more often than not I continued to steer my own raft down the most difficult parts of the river, because I didn't know the river. I didn't understand the dangers of the river; yet I was insistent upon following my own map, packing my own supplies, and doing everything my way.

The greatest gift born from my cancer was this newfound awareness of and perspective on life. I can clearly see that if I had only allowed God to guide my raft down the river, the journey would have been so much smoother. Sometimes no matter which fork you take in the river, you are going to hit rough waters; but when God is guiding the raft, even the roughest of waters become much easier to navigate. If only someone had told me this in my twenties! Trust in the Lord, and He will get you through the roughest parts of your life—that is faith.

Clearly putting trust in the Lord is a part of faith. It is so simple yet quite often overlooked. Yes, in order to have faith we must believe. But two people can believe in God's existence equally—yet one has stronger faith because they put more trust in God to guide their journey than the other who, say, continuously tries to impose their own will along the journey.

I used to be the "other" in that scenario. I believed, but I couldn't see (I was blind, but now I see) that my faith was lacking. My own stubbornness and pride played a giant role in my misguided path, which ultimately led me to nothing other than disappointment, stress, restlessness, and brain cancer—all brought upon me by me trying to impose my will upon this world rather than simply trusting

God to guide the way. We need Him and even more so when we have cancer! Yes, I blame myself, not God, not science, but me (for acquiring cancer). It is not my intention to make you feel like your cancer is your fault, not at all. My story is unique, and I will get to it in the third chapter.

My friends, I can (and later on in this book I will) personally attest to the grace and many blessings I've received from God since I placed all my trust in Him.

I thought I had faith before, but in retrospect I did not even understand what faith actually was.

I believed in God, but I didn't have a relationship with Him. The heavenly Father wants you to have a relationship with Him but even more so with His beloved Son, Jesus Christ. "Jesus said to him, I am the Way, and the Truth and the Life; no one comes to the Father but through Me" (John 14:6).

If you don't already, I encourage you to start talking to Christ every day! Before you begin this life-changing journey, allow me to offer a few dos and don'ts.

Please do not spit your verbal diarrhea at Jesus. Nobody wants their brother to constantly whine and beg them for things. And don't barter with God—"God, if You do this, I promise that from now on I'll always…" Stop. There's nothing you can do for God that He couldn't do for you a trillion times over, so please…no bartering. God expects you to try your best to live free of sin, and so it is an expectation, not a bargaining chip.

Start your prayer life by getting to know Him. Build that relationship, and He will hear you. Just talk to Jesus, and more importantly spend time in silence with and listening to Him. Jesus desires to have a relationship with every one of us; after all He did die on the cross for each and every one of us.

The difference between those two segments of the same notion of faith made a staggering difference in my life once I figured it out, and it can do the same for you.

You see, I believe in my mother; but if I didn't have a relationship with her, I sure wouldn't place a lot of trust in her. But because I have a relationship with my mom and therefore know she has a brilliant medical mind, I tend to place a lot of trust in her when it comes to not only medical advice but other things as well. Out of that relationship grows a degree of trust; and you can have that same relationship with God, Jesus Christ, and the Holy Spirit once you come to know Them by taking the time to do so. All you have to do is carve out some time to talk to Him every day. More importantly, spend time in silence listening to Him. There are references in the Bible to being still before God.

We want God to speak with us as humans do. I used to believe that too, but not anymore. If God acted like a human, how disappointing would that be? He wouldn't be all wise. He would not be wise at all. His heart would be wicked. I want God to act godly.

So I offer you this:

> *Be still before the Lord and wait patiently for Him. (Psalm 37:7)*

CHAPTER 2

Bolstering Your Belief

Having to defend the Christian faith gives more plausibility to its dissenters than they even deserve, so I don't wish to spend much time here. With that being said, we—as Christians—should all prepare ourselves to be able to defend our faith. And I will bravely swim the waters of political correctness here, defending it against atheists, agnostics, Muslims, Hindus, and those who bitterly wave their finger at the sky blaming a god they don't even believe in for all their problems and iniquities.

Christianity is a faith that, for the record, has more evidence to support it than it does to denounce it, more so than any other worldview or religion.

It is not my intention to assail any other worldviews, but nor will I cower from my convictions to appease the delicate sensibilities of those who would persecute me. Haven't we all learned by now that our so-called cultural *tolerance* is abhorrently *intolerant*? I will not deny my Lord Jesus Christ Who said, "Whosoever shall deny me before men, him will I also deny before my Father who is in heaven" (Matthew 10:33).

I have many friends whom I love, who happen to hold other worldviews. I have come to love all of mankind, but I can disagree and love simultaneously! This simple ability should *not* be viewed as insoluble because in doing so we are taking giant leaps backward as a species. Redirecting while disrespecting someone's worldview is a direct path to regression. It is a simple, logical notion that is tragically disappearing from our society.

Pride and vanity are the chief causes for which a person tends to become hateful toward others whom they cannot impose their own beliefs upon, and I would encourage such people to undergo a deep self-reflection and discover how they have come to live such a hateful existence.

I no longer waste time and energy arguing with those people. I use that time instead to pray for them.

It was the late, brilliant Christian apologetic Ravi Zacharias who said to those people he loved who could not accept God's moral laws, "God has given you the most gracious gift of the prerogative of choice, but God does not give you the privilege of determining a different outcome of what that choice will entail."

Here is merely one example I will give you to get you prepared to defend your faith against some of the biggest opposition, and then we will move on because this topic could be its own book; and if you search for a book on this subject, you can find many.

As Christians you will hear dissenters from all over the world shoving the theory of evolution in your face as they laugh at you for believing in God. That's okay. Simply ask them then to explain their worldview, which must replace yours. If they cannot produce one, then you can point out that their opposition to your worldview is irrelevant because it does nothing to disprove or replace yours.

If they give you evolution as a substitute, then simply point them to their own brilliant scientists Wickramasinghe and Hoyle who wrote the book *Evolution from Space*. In the book they had to conclude that "The mathematical responsibility of the protein formulation is impossible to explain in an earthbound theory."

Based on that conclusion, and using their stubbornness for ignoring theism, they developed what is called the panspermia theory. Essentially this theory proposes that spores from another planet came to seed the earth. Okay, well, how about the rest of the universe from which these spores supposedly were derived? (I'm shrugging my shoulders.)

I know. I know. But there are people who would rather believe in alien spores than a divine creator. To me it is laughable when these wonderful people call us Christians "the gullible ones."

Strap in, folks. I'll do you one better here. A brilliant quantum physicist (John Polkinghorne) from Cambridge University concurred that if you would take the expansion and contraction rates needed to create our universe, the exactitude demanded was so perfect and the margin of error so small that if it had been one picosecond off, it would have collapsed.

Then he created an analogy: if you were to take aim at a square inch object, twenty *billion* light-years away, you would have to have hit it bull's-eye to create our universe.

I suppose then that we gullible Christians can conclude that God, aside from being all-powerful and intelligent, is also a pretty good shot.

The intelligence demanded behind the creation of our universe supports a creator! Otherwise, we are merely the product of time plus matter plus *extreme* chance. Okay then, but don't call me gullible for believing in God, you little alien sperm, you (wink, wink).

I gathered this information from minds far more brilliant than mine, and you can certainly research it all in far more depth on your own. But if that doesn't make you look a little more toward the heavens, folks, then I'm not sure what will do it.

Okay, are we feeling a little more secure with God's existence? Then let's move on to even more challenging issues surrounding our faith so that we may move beyond them and get on with battling our cancer strongly in faith with Christ on our side.

CHAPTER 3

Developing a Relationship with Christ

I have good news for you: this is not a difficult thing to achieve *if* you desire it. I can't make you desire it though—that's the catch. You have to desire in your heart to have a relationship with Christ.

A suggestion for those of you who do not feel the desire would be to attend a few churches and see if you can find a pastor or a priest who speaks a message straight into your heart. Another thing to do would be to watch the series *The Chosen*, one of my favorite visual stories about Christ. See if that doesn't enflame your desire to come to know Christ.

I believe that on some level we all do. We are drawn to the Creator, our soul to His spirit, and we remain restless on earth and unfulfilled until we realize what it is that we are truly seeking—the very thing from which we came, God.

And how do you get to the Father? Through the Son. Start talking to Jesus every day. Read the Gospels and see what He has already spoken to us. Put aside a few moments of your day to sit in silence with Him.

If you are new to prayer, the idea is not to be distracted by your surroundings so that you may focus. Let me give you an idea on how to get started. The most powerful conversation I ever had with Christ began in this way: sitting in a Catholic church in adoration before the Eucharist. But you can accomplish this anywhere in silence.

Begin by sharing a few things with Jesus that you are excited about and grateful for (speak to Him as you would a close friend) and then go on to share a few concerns you have. Ask Jesus to place those worries in the Father's hands and then simply enjoy His peace in silence as you listen.

This is how your faith can grow. Eventually you will feel His presence if you ask Him for it enough. Depending on your current strength of faith, this might happen immediately, or it might take some time. But it will happen. Do not allow yourself to become so discouraged that you stop talking to God. Even when you think He is not listening, one day something will happen in your life that will confirm that, indeed, God was listening the entire time. The solution or answer may not be the one you wanted or expected. Keep listening to Him.

Every morning I literally just sit down for a second and ask God, "Let me feel Your presence and Your peace today, Lord."

The first time I underwent a radiation treatment on my brain, I begged Jesus to go with me. I was undoubtedly concerned though I tried not to show it. But even when others around me couldn't tell how afraid I was, Jesus knew.

They placed the mask over my face, which they had molded specifically for me, and bolted it to the table. I'm not kidding you. It was like something out of a horror film, and it brought about the oddest feeling of claustrophobia I had ever experienced in my life. I remember thinking, perhaps even out loud—I cannot recall—*Lord, how did it come to this?*

Almost instantly I felt a calm overtake my body even though I was as nervous as I'd ever been.

The machine began to move, and as I gazed into the only direction in which I could (up), the red light on the machine that fixated my vision was in the shape of a cross. I see that same red cross every time I get an MRI. I still don't know if it was designed that way for a scientific reason or if the designer had guidance from the divine or if it's just what I see.

The moment I stared into that red cross, I felt Jesus's presence in that room. I asked Him to take my hand, and He did. Throughout the next forty-some treatments, I felt His presence with me in that room every single time.

How did my relationship with Christ begin? Prayer. Is it so unfathomable to think that the Lord Jesus Christ wants to get to know you? Of course He does! He loves us more than we can possibly understand. Can we fully comprehend a divine love? The Greeks call it agape, the highest form of love imaginable.

Listen to me, friend. If you can't give Christ a few minutes of your time every day to get to know Him, then you can't expect Him to be in that room with you.

If you set aside time every day to speak with Jesus Christ, I promise you that your life will begin to change for the better. Just make the effort. If you can give two minutes, then give two minutes. If you can give ten minutes, then give ten.

I talk to God all day long. While I'm in the shower, driving in my car, or having a meal, He's always on my mind. He's always with me. I also set aside time every morning to meet with Him, and this is where my most powerful prayer typically happens.

Honestly, because of this prayer life, I live mostly free from fear. Although I have the deadliest form of brain cancer there is, I live a fairly "normal" life. The truth is I hardly ever think about brain cancer because I put that concern in God's hands.

It was not always like this for me—not until I started taking the time to have a relationship with Jesus Christ. Looking back on my life now, it's easy for me to extrapolate this sense that He was always with me. I had simply failed to acknowledge Him.

It's like we were both in the same cafeteria, but He was sitting at the table in front of me patting the seat beside Him, inviting me to come and sit. My overly busy, overly caffeinated mind was unable to take notice of Him through the fog of my own concerns and aspirations. How foolish it was to leave Him out of those things.

He always loved me. Now that I've gotten to know Jesus, I love Him, and we have a relationship of brotherhood, acknowledging the same heavenly Father. Of course, He is the only begotten Son of God, and I am merely human, but Jesus is indeed our brother.

I urge you to begin your relationship with Christ right now. Set this book down and talk with Jesus Christ for a few minutes. Give Him just a slice of your time, a piece of recognition in this moment, and see what happens. That is far more important than anything else I've written in this book.

CHAPTER 4

God Works through People

Let me properly welcome you to the family! I know. I know…the family you never wanted, my exact thoughts when my mother gave me a sealed folder containing a letter from another guy around my age who had been fighting the same type of brain cancer as me for years. The first line of the letter, or even the heading perhaps, said, "Welcome to the family."

I sealed that file back up and would not open it again for months to come. I wasn't excited about having a cancer family. Let me tell you friends with assuredness that I am overly blessed today to have this cancer family.

You cannot take on this beast by yourself. Some people are more receptive to taking an outstretched hand than others. However, in the case that you are a stubborn, prideful individual as I once was who does not like taking "handouts," get over yourself for your own sake.

You cannot win this battle alone. The wonderful thing about cancer is that you have so many resources available to you. The awareness of and support for cancer have grown tremendously in the last decade alone. As strange as it sounds, there has never been a better time in all of history for you to have cancer than right now.

You are going to face new physical, emotional, and financial challenges all because of cancer. I'm here to tell you there is a lot of support out there to help you overcome all these things! Now, do not be so foolish as to say to me, "But I'm just going to put this in God's hands, right?"

God works through people. He always has. If you believe Jesus Christ is the Son of God, then you believe Jesus is God, and Jesus sent men and women out to do His work before returning to be seated at the right hand of the Father in heaven.

Yes, *women too.* There are plenty of examples of God working through women in the Bible. Mary Magdalene was a disciple of Christ, and I don't think that's really debatable. God worked through our Holy Mother Mary to come into the world so He could redeem us!

There are plenty of other examples of God working through women in the Bible: Ruth, Rachel, Ezra, Deborah, Miriam, Sarah, Esther, and so on. Not to mention all the wonderful female saints we have had or have. I felt the importance to point this out for those of you who were not privy to it, and I'll leave it at that. I have actually heard women call the church sexist. You are going to the wrong church if you feel this way, and you probably need to find a new priest or pastor.

God does so much of His work through people. So pray for the doctors performing surgeries on and treating cancer patients; pray for the scientists working hard on finding better treatments and cures; pray for all the social workers and wonderful organizations that help to fund these endeavors and those who seek to relieve our physical, emotional, and financial burdens as cancer patients. Pray that the Holy Spirit might work through them and place your trust in God.

CHAPTER 5

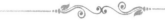

Focus on Your Fight

We all have difficult questions, more so when you get that diagnosis—the who, the what, the why, the how. Even as someone who believes so deeply in the Father, the Son, and the Holy Spirit, I still have questions.

Jesus Christ gave us so many of those answers in the Gospels if you take the time to read them and furthermore allow a spiritual advisor or a Christian theologian to help you interpret Christ's messages.

I'm always willing to learn more, anxious even. Have you ever thought about what you might ask Christ or the Father when you meet Him? I certainly have. But with time I've come to realize that I am more afraid of what He might ask me than I am concerned about what I might ask Him.

When you are diagnosed with something as horrific as cancer, these questions go from universal to very centrically focused on your situation—as they should. The concerns of the world are no longer your concerns. You need to leave those concerns to God's healthy children and focus on your fight—at least until you get better.

Maybe before cancer you were a staunch environmentalist fighting climate change, or perhaps you were involved heavily in politics protesting for justice or obsessed with bringing clean water to certain parts of the world. Maybe you were very career centric.

Listen to me: those concerns are no longer yours. If you don't focus on your health and getting better, what more can you offer on this earth once you're buried within it? Worrying about these things will only cause you to stress.

Stress is the number one enemy of a cancer patient. There are many studies (and my personal experience) clearly demonstrating a direct correlation between chronic stress and cancer.

When you are stressed, neurotransmitters are released that can actually stimulate cancer cells; and if you are already battling cancer, then you'd better not be riling up the enemy. In part 2 of this book, I will give you some tips on how to battle stress.

You might be currently stuck thinking thoughts such as *God, how could You let this happen to me? What did I do to deserve this? Why me?*

These types of thoughts actually inhibit you from overcoming stress.

That being said, they are all fair questions, the bulk of which I hope I can help you address in the following chapters so that you might move forward into a positive relationship with the Lord.

This is a tough subject to tackle, so pray for me. Pray for us. Just know that I've read into some of the brightest minds there are on this subject, so you're in good hands. I'm not just making this stuff up based on a feeling or a bias. Whether you have been recently diagnosed with cancer or hit by a car, lost a spouse, or suffered a miscarriage, it all comes down to suffering. God, why do we suffer?

CHAPTER 6

Intro to Faith and Suffering

God is all wise, and humans are certainly not. Therefore, we have a difficult time finding reason within certain parameters. That being said I cannot simply tell you to trust God at this intersect as that directive feels a bit lackluster when we are discussing something like suffering with cancer. So why all this pain and suffering?

This is a vast topic that has been debated and explained in church teachings for a long time. I would like to segue into this with one of my favorite analogies.

When I was young (and I'm sure you can recall similar experiences), my mother took me to a doctor's office and allowed some strange woman to stab me with a pointy metal object that caused physical pain. I remember feeling a slight anguish toward my mother. "How could she let this happen if she loved me?"

Now that I'm a father and have a son who is deathly afraid of needles, I understand the why of this situation in a much deeper context. It was out of *love* that she had me subjected to this pain because of course the vaccine would save me from far worse pain and suffering later on in life. Every time I have to take my needle-phobic son in for a vaccine, I feel just awful because I know how frightened he is going to be; and it's hard for me to watch, but I know it is for his own good.

But try explaining this to a small child. See if you can get them to believe you're about to let some stranger stab them and it's all because you love them. We are God's children. Do you understand how this correlates?

God indeed works in mysterious ways, and we have no way of completely deciphering His divine wisdom; but perhaps we can, with time, draw closer to an understanding.

All will be revealed to us in the end, and many of us will probably have a jaw-dropping experience as we react, "Ohhhhh, yes... I understand now. Thank You, God!"

In the meantime, let us try to make *some* sense out of this while we are stuck here with our feeble human minds, which in my opinion is better than playing the blame game and carrying around bitterness. It is most certainly better for your health.

We carry this notion with us from the time we are small children that if you do good, you'll be rewarded and if you do bad, you will be punished. In religious terms we tend to apply this same notion as if you do bad things, you will be cursed and if you do good things, you will be blessed. Be careful with that. Sometimes what is "good" for us and what is "bad" for us get jumbled and mixed up in our human understanding and emotions.

I believe it was harder for my mother to watch me suffer the pain of that needle than it was for me to actually endure the pain. This is the same with me and my son. God's love for His children is even greater, and He proved that through Jesus Christ. God does not enjoy watching us suffer, but He is leading us on a journey, and it is impossible to reach our final destination without suffering as Christ did.

Can you imagine how hard it must be for God to watch us suffer and stumble through this world? Just because we do not understand doesn't mean that God does not understand. We would do well to remember that God is love.

CHAPTER 7

Take Up Your Cancer Cross

Then Jesus told His disciples, "If anyone would come after me, let him deny himself and take up his cross and follow me. For whoever would save his life will lose it, but whoever loses his life for my sake will find it. For what will profit a man if he gains the whole world and forfeits his soul? Or what shall a man give in return for his soul?" (Matthew 16:24–26).

I refuse to leave you hanging here. Let's decipher this most important message from Jesus together. I am not sure there is anything more powerful than these words for those of us carrying our cancer cross.

In the very first line, Jesus is telling us if we want redemption, if we want to enter the kingdom of heaven one day, which of course we are all being called toward, then we must give up our own sinful earthly wants and desires. Now, to take up our cross literally means we will suffer. The only way to redemption is through suffering. Jesus suffered on the cross to redeem us all, and He is merely handing us a sliver of that cross to carry so that we may bring His sacrifice to fruition by following Him regardless of the cost. If He is not the most important thing in your life, then you will not find eternal life.

The next line speaks about whoever loses their life for Jesus will find eternal life. But if you choose to make your life easier on this fallen-from-grace earth by denying Him and knowingly partaking in sin (which will never lead to happiness by the way), you will lose your life. He means your eternal life. Thus, your soul will be lost from God. But if you live your life for Christ and follow in His ways while forsaking your own, you will enter the kingdom of heaven.

The following lines are my favorite:

> *For what will profit a man if he gains the whole world and forfeits his soul? Or what shall a man give in return for his soul?*

The first line reminds me of a man named Jordan Belfort, whom you may be familiar with from either his memoir or the blockbuster film starring Leonardo DiCaprio, *The Wolf of Wall Street.*

Jordan Belfort lived a life we most likely never will. He lived in lavish beyond our grasp. He enjoyed the finest riches this earth has to offer and lived in exquisite comfort. It might all seem incredible and even desirable to us. Our culture certainly promotes it. Think about what Jordan Belfort had to give up for all that…his soul.

> *Do not store up for yourselves treasures on earth, where moth and rust destroy and where thieves break in and steal, but lay up for yourselves treasures in heaven where neither moth nor rust destroys and where thieves do not break in and steal. For where your treasure is, there your heart will be also. (Matthew 6:19–21)*

Belfort cheated so many innocent people out of money by tricking them into buying into his "pump and dump" scams. Some of these people were persuaded to give every saved penny they had, led to believe that their little pot of nickels could be turned into a pot of gold, all fraudulently of course.

The final line poses a question:

> *Or what shall a man give in return for his soul?*

There is nothing we can give God to buy our soul back once our time is up. That is it. Game over. You either pick up your cross on earth and suffer with Christ, or you give up your soul, and what can you give in return for that?

I must add that I have no idea as to the current state of Jordan Belfort's soul. I hope for his sake that he has repented and renounced greed since serving his prison sentence. He is a child of God, and ergo God desires him to come to Him in heaven too. But it seems greed is his cross to bear, something God has obviously given him to overcome.

Remember, my friends, our life on earth is merely the journey, not the destination. We are all called back to that from which we came, to God the Creator.

Our cross to bear is something we must overcome! I did not understand why God gave me cancer, but something inside me knew better than to turn bitter against Him and instead simply turn toward Him. The more I turn to Him, the better my life gets, and that is the truth.

This is His intention. We suffer to be reminded that we need to turn to God. Let us not forsake and forget our God. History has shown worldly consequences again and again of those who move further from God and/or worship false gods.

So now, my friends, I invite you to pick up your cancer cross and turn toward the Lord with me.

You have cancer, but you are not dead. Let us store up our treasures in heaven and get to know Christ better today. So when we knock on that gate at the end of the narrow path, Christ will recognize us and welcome us into His kingdom with a warm embrace.

CHAPTER 8

Deeper into Suffering

To really understand what we are going through, it is crucial that we understand suffering as much as we can while retaining our faith. If I didn't feel it was important, I would have gladly skipped over this dreary topic and moved directly into other forums of fighting with faith.

I promise you that this book will not leave you feeling gloomy if you can "suffer" through it (insert bad joke). Yet even in how we come to look at a seemingly dire topic such as suffering, when brought into a meaningful perspective, it sheds layers of darkness and begins to appear brighter for us. This is the love and mercy of God.

During my studies in college, I had a particular professor I was fond of. She was, however, a self-proclaimed atheist. I still loved her and the many wonderful qualities that she possessed. I never considered her to be a bad person at all.

But she would, on occasion, say things like "How could God let a hurricane wipe out so many people?" I had no answers for her back then. I just sat in silence feeling as though I had been attacked and was unable to defend myself. Following Christ is not easy; but I know what I will gain by doing so. I have since studied my faith in much further depth (thereby strengthening my faith), and so I will now respond to that professor's inquiry.

My initial response to her would be to say that an atheist really has no right to ask that question because it is not a moral framework that they operate within. The atheist has no philosophical base on which to ask the question. The Hindu doesn't ask it because to them it must be karma, and the Muslim simply says, "It is the will of God." The Buddhist would say, "They are all being born again through samsara" or "They have achieved nirvana and suffer no more."

So if you are legitimizing the question, then you are simultaneously legitimizing the Judeo-Christian worldview. Otherwise, it is an illegitimate question. I say to you now, Professor, thank you for legitimizing my worldview.

Now we can answer her question from within that paradigm—the paradigm of God's creation and purpose. Humanity's violation of that purpose offers the entailments of that purpose, which are internal brokenness (cancer/disease), external brokenness, and brokenness in relation to the elements and the powers that are around us (natural disasters, war). He warned us this would happen and in fact tells us that during the end of times the occurrences of these will increase along with wars and the rumors of wars.

Here it is: God created us with purpose and design. We broke that purpose and design, and now we reap the consequences all around and within us.

In the midst of these tragedies, it is our responsibility to reach out to others with the love of Christ to keep hearts from hardening. We do not stand back and watch it happen and let our hearts grow bitter. My small hometown recently underwent a devastating flood, and it was truly inspiring to see people come together and help one another through the aftermath of the crisis.

I was not personally affected, but some of my friends unfortunately were. My sons and I went into the disaster zone and hauled damage out of the area for people so they could begin to rebuild their homes and their lives. Because I own a truck, this is how I was able to help.

Out of this devastation I saw the scorn of a bitter person who posted on Facebook asking, "Where was God during this flood?" In the comment section below that, I read a brilliant response that made me smile. The response read as such:

> *As devastating as this was to our community, in the wake of such loss, homes being completely swept away, an entire town gone underwater, there were zero deaths. So, to answer your question, God was busy saving lives.*

Now hold on a minute before you bushwhack me; I realize that many natural disasters do incur deaths. If you pose the question, then you are legitimizing the Judeo-Christian worldview, and it may not be the answer we desire. But put shortly God didn't bring this devastation upon mankind. We are a fallen species, and we have to reap that which we have sown, but through God's love and mercy He can and will raise us up!

Do not live for this world. Do not store up your treasures on earth. Store up your treasures in heaven, for you never know when disaster will strike you down.

If you walk in the ways of Christ, then just like Christ you too can conquer death. That is the redemption He offers, and it is in this alone that you may or may not take your final breaths in solace.

Peel back the layers of darkness, my friends. Christ's suffering on the cross led to His triumph over death itself. Pick up your cross, take courage, and fight your cancer with faith. Contemplate on what you have gained from this disease rather than what you have lost.

Thus is the love and mercy of God. In order to experience this love and mercy, you need to enter a relationship with Jesus Christ. You are still breathing, my friends, so you have not failed!

PART 2

How Do I Get By?

CHAPTER 9

Resources

N ow with a better understanding of why we suffer while remaining in a positive coherence with God, let us move forward with hope, faith, and love.

Allow me now to welcome you to the family! I know it is not a cancer family you desire, but it is a cancer family you have. Let me assure you that it is a very supportive family, and if you know where to look, you will be overwhelmed with the generosity and support you receive from people who truly wish to help you, people God called on to help you.

It is time for you to open up to the idea of receiving help. If you are anything like I was, then your pride might be getting in the way of your thrive. Essentially, in order to thrive, you must throw out your pride. You are not the same person you were if you are currently undergoing treatment for cancer. Major surgeries, chemo, and radiation all take their toll on us.

I will address this quickly: For those of you who may have been biopsied, been diagnosed, and had your cancer surgically removed with little fear of it ever returning, good for you, brothers and sisters! I am overjoyed for you. With that said, this chapter is probably not meant for you.

For those of you in the thick of the battle, here are some important things for you to know.

First of all, almost every major county has some sort of a Cancer Services office. In my county in Michigan, it is literally called Cancer Services. I can almost guarantee that you have something similar nearby. In Lincoln, Nebraska, it is called the CTCA. In Burlington, Vermont, it is called the UVM Cancer Center. Beyond these localized support offices, organizations like the American Cancer Society operate all over—you guessed it—America.

I'll never forget the day I received a random phone call from a caseworker who introduced herself with a Cancer Services affiliation. Immediately, my heart sank. Anytime cancer patients receive a phone call and hear the word *cancer*, we can't help but suffer through a miniature heart attack wondering, *Oh no…is my cancer back?* or *Is this another bill I can't afford?* It is precisely that feeling of "My Lord, what must I bear now?" Even for the most pious of people, it can be hard to suppress this initial reaction to that word, *cancer*.

Fortuitously for me, the call was from a case manager who worked at my local Cancer Services office. She had received my information from a friend of my mother who just happened to personally know this particular caseworker and thought she might be able to help me somehow.

I am not sure I ever would have found them on my own. I didn't know anything about Cancer Services, and I had never been close enough to someone who had cancer to experience that journey with them—in short, I was clueless.

God knows what we need. I happened to be at a point in my journey where I was starting to think I'd like to meet others with cancer outside of the hospital setting to see if I could help them in any way. I wanted to give back after all the help I'd received from amazing friends and family.

My strength and energy were returning somewhat (though never fully), and I had this almost innate desire to help others in any way possible.

The case manager told me about several ways in which they could help *me*. Wait. Help me? Why?

I thought I had everything I needed already, but my presumption could not have been further from reality. Some of the worst things about being a continuous cancer patient are the never-ending bills, the constant battle with insurance... Heck, I even had the government coming after me for student loans wanting to take my disability income away from me as I was not even employed at that time.

I was living on disability scraps, and everyone was trying to take the pieces. I have two sons who live with me, and we were trying to survive on that. "I thought you were married and had a normal life?" you ask. Yes, well, I underwent an extremely disheartening divorce six months after my diagnosis. I'll dive into that delightfulness later.

Through the judiciary system, it was determined that my sons were to move 150 miles north (from where I'd been living as a married man) with me and attend school (in the small town where all my family lives). Thus, during the school year, the children primarily live with me.

These financial hardships are very real for many of us fighting cancer. They were certainly hitting me from all sides, and just when I solved one dilemma, it seemed another would quickly arise. And we all know stress is the enemy.

That phone call from Cancer Services changed my life. They were able to unravel many of the issues I was facing. Furthermore, they directed me toward organizations that would resolve other issues that they could not directly address themselves.

Find them. Find your nearest Cancer Services office. You will not regret it. You should not have to fight cancer and insurance companies and pharmacies and the government all at once. I swear sometimes it felt as though they were all trying to kill me. I would be remiss if I failed to admit that oftentimes I felt perhaps it would be easier to simply give in and to die already.

Of course, that mental framework is extremely selfish. Yes, you read that properly, S-E-L-F-I-S-H! I have two sons who need me, family and friends who love me, and a lot to offer this world before I take my rightful place bowed down at the feet of my merciful Lord.

If you just read the previous paragraph and said to yourself, "I don't have those things," then to you I say you are still breathing and it is not too late for you to start living. Begin by putting other people first. Form some meaningful relationships, and I'm not alluding to romance. Friendship can be so much more powerful than that. You don't have a loving, supporting family? Build one. It can start right at your local Cancer Services center, or it can start at your church. It's out there. The bottom line is: there is a reason that you are still here. You must discover that reason through prayer. Do not squander this second chance you've been given. It might be that you have been granted some more time to come to know the Lord. There may even be another purpose He created you for that you have yet to fulfill. It would bring my heart great joy to know that reading this book helped you to discover that.

My Cancer Services center holds monthly group meetings for all local cancer patients/survivors, as well as hosting special group events by age that are unique and fun. I've met some great new friends from attending these events.

My local Cancer Services center also helps with travel expenses for treatments by distributing gas cards and gift cards to restaurants as needed. I was traveling two-and-a-half hours every couple of months for testing and checkups, and this really helped take some financial stress away from those already stressful trips.

Thanks to the generosity of Cancer Services, I have been able to explore and come to benefit from many other services I otherwise never would have, such as counseling, meditation, and even some unique treatments like Reiki. One of the coolest things to ever happen to me is when I was sent on an all-expenses-paid cruise with my sons by the Megan Mae Foundation! My sons still rave about that trip. It was Cancer Services who gave the foundation my information. Elsewise, they might not have found me.

Cancer Services also referred me to another organization in my town (otherwise nonexistent to me) known as the Pardee Cancer Treatment Fund. Before my dealings with Pardee, I absolutely dreaded going to my mailbox. My medical bills would cause a middle-class man stroke and make an upper-class man curse out loud.

Now, thanks to Pardee, every time I get some inconceivable medical bill, a bill that *most people* couldn't afford, I simply have to forward the bill to them and they take care of it.

Aside from the obvious benefit of not having my credit score implode due to ghastly medical bills, this has removed a huge amount of stress from my life and has added years to it, and years are priceless to a cancer warrior.

I encourage you, I implore you, and I beg you to find your nearest Cancer Services center and speak with a caseworker.

There are also social workers in most hospitals who can often help relieve your financial burdens. Someone who works at the hospital wherein I was first admitted and treated found a company to cover what my insurance will not (a grotesque number) for the medical device that I wear. Without them, I would *not* be able to afford to wear the device, without which I don't know if I'd still be here or not.

Listen to me again, please. Your stress level affects your physical health. Financial stress can be devastating for cancer patients.

I have a magic eight ball analogy. Since coming to work with Cancer Services and other similar organizations, the quality of my life went from "outlook not so good" to "outlook good." No exaggerations.

You need to shed as many layers of financial stress, emotional stress, and physical stress as you possibly can! Remember the world's problems are no longer your problems. Focus on your health.

God understood my needs, and so it was no coincidence when the Holy Spirit whispered my name into the ear of a family friend at the right moment in time, and in turn she gave it to the caseworker at Cancer Services. Trust me I had been praying for God to help me with these issues long before I received that phone call.

Aside from the financial stress relief, another benefit from Cancer Services has been all the wonderful people I've met as a result of this affiliation.

It is incredibly beneficial to make friends with others who are fighting this beast as it takes away feelings of isolation. Any notions you might carry of "Why me?" will assuredly dissipate when you meet other wonderful people who are also carrying this cross. If that doesn't at least turn your "Why me?" into a "Why them?" then might I suggest to you without being facetious that you do some deep self-reflection concerning that.

Meeting others with cancer also provides you with people to speak with whom you can relate to and seek advice from. Priceless. I have attained hoards of advice from other cancer warriors when I opened up to them about some of my hardships, and in return they told me how they were able to overcome the same obstacles.

God works through people. Cancer Services has led me to multiple organizations who all help cancer patients in unique ways. Find them. God chose these people to help with your afflictions. Arguing with God is a frivolous exercise. (I know all too well from my days of playing tour guide over my own life.) Find these wonderful people and let them do what God has called them to do.

If you're unsure where to turn, ask your doctor to put you in touch with one of the hospital's social workers. (I believe most hospitals have them.) That's a great place to start.

CHAPTER 10

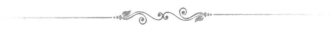

Approach to Anxiety

There is no single approach to anxiety, and there's no magic switch to turn it off. Sorry to be the bearer of bad news. There is no way to cease worrying entirely, especially as a cancer warrior. Every time a new scan date approaches, we feel at a minimum slight apprehension.

Your concerns are natural, and they are meant to turn you to the Lord! He has so many designs for getting us to notice Him, and it is extremely unfortunate when so many of us miss these.

Let us differentiate here between Merriam-Webster's two main collegiate definitions for anxiety:

1. Apprehensive uneasiness or nervousness usually over an impending or anticipated ill: a state of being anxious
2. *Medical:* an abnormal and overwhelming sense of apprehension and fear often marked by physical signs (such as tension, sweating, and increased pulse rate), by doubt concerning the reality and nature of the threat, and by self-doubt about one's capacity to cope with it

We all suffer from the first type, with or without cancer. As human beings we are supposed to from time to time. Look at it as more of a super sense, if you will.

I am walking to my car parked down the street in the dark. *I don't remember parking so far down. I begin to feel uneasy, a bit nervous as if something wasn't right. I hear a strange noise. I see movement where there should be none.*

In this state of being, your senses actually do heighten, and whether there is a bogeyman looming in a bush may or may not (hopefully) be the case. Either way your chances of survival are elevated because of your anxiety. If someone does jump out at you, you will be quicker to take notice because you are in an anxious state of being, and that can improve your reaction time and thereby your odds of escaping.

When you are fighting cancer, the threat is always there. The bogeyman is always looming in the bush. It's just a matter of if/when he will strike again.

Herein lies the question, which thereby poses the potential problem: is your level of anxiety typical or medical? Either way, you are suffering, and so you must turn to God for help of course. Ask Jesus what you should do. It might be that you just need to learn to put more trust in Him; or you might be suffering from medical anxiety, which can present physical symptoms actually taxing to your health (stress = cancer's number one ally). But which one is yours?

As I clearly stated in the introduction, I am not a medical expert, but I have studied the issue of anxiety and know a few people who do suffer or have suffered from it on a medical level.

If you are headed to a treatment appointment or a scan to see whether or not your cancer is returning, it is absolutely natural for you to feel anxious.

If, however, your anxiety feels unmanageable (even after prayer) and you are feeling physical symptoms, such as dizziness, rapid heartbeat, shortness of breath, tingling in the extremities, and so on, but your test result comes back clean, do you now find yourself doubting the good test results? When positive news has no impact on lowering or decimating said anxiety, then chances are you have a medical/mental health issue with anxiety, my friend. Please discuss the issue with your doctor. I have two friends who are on prescriptions for anxiety, without which they could not even function normally on a daily basis.

Do you find yourself not doing things in your life you would normally do because your anxiety scares you so much?

Ask yourself if you experience this type of thoughts: *If I go for a jog, I might pass out in the street and get run over. I need to cancel my plans with friends today so they don't see my anxiety. I need to back out of this trip because I could embarrass myself by having heart palpitations in front of people. My odds are better of surviving today if I simply lie here in bed.*

This paragraph is important to read: Your current physical state of being or perhaps your medications may hinder your capabilities. You may have a list of things your doctor recommends you should not do. Be careful not to confuse these things you are not supposed to do with symptoms of medical anxiety.

Do not feel embarrassed if you believe you are suffering from medical anxiety. Seek help because you may have a real problem. It can be difficult to decipher in our modern-day culture, I know.

We live in a society where people record videos of themselves having "panic attacks" and post them online. They usually make some type of claim before or after that "panic attacks are real." Some of these might be real, but some of them overshadow a real crisis with self-victimization and attention-seeking behavior.

Bottom line: Anxiety and depression can be very real and serious issues and hence a personal problem that should be dealt with personally. "When you pray, do not be like the hypocrites who love to pray publicly on street corners and in the synagogues where everyone can see them. I tell you the truth, that is all the reward they will ever get" (Matthew 6:5).

I believe this principle holds true for all those people who victimize themselves on social media as well, craving pity for themselves, while people with real problems are praying to God behind closed doors, refusing to be a victim and instead being warriors.

Be a cancer warrior, not a cancer victim, for it is truly the only mindset that prevails in this battle.

Sorry if that seems harsh, but this book after all is called *Fighting with Faith*. It is *not* called *Fighting with Facebook*. Although I cannot deny the ability of social media to raise awareness and perhaps offer you some much needed help in the process, allow me to clearly state that I'm only speaking on your use of social media in regard to the context of your mindset.

If you are experiencing a "typical" level of anxiety (which is probably a bit higher for us cancer folks), then prayer is your number one tool to combat the issue. The Bible tells us 365 times to not be afraid, one time for every single day of the year. You think maybe God was really trying to drive this point home? Turn to Him, place your worries in His hands, offer up your sufferings for the sake of others, take courage, and fear not—all messages from the Bible.

I've always considered myself to be an extremely mentally/emotionally strong individual, easily able to determine factual from fictional anxiety, but even I have suffered from it. It is unavoidable.

Stop: More to that story.

This just happened to me while writing about medical anxiety in this book. Strange, but true.

I just recently suffered through a violent seizure, probably the scariest thing I have ever experienced in my life. My heart goes out to people who suffer from these frequently.

I experienced so much anxiety after the seizure that it literally changed my life. I stopped playing guitar (a passion of mine) because it happened while I was playing. Fortunately, I had a minor premonition seconds before that something was wrong and was able to set the guitar aside and lie down on the floor prior to the grand mal seizure.

I had no control as the left side of my body convulsed violently and my left arm in particular flailed wildly. The left side of my face felt like it was warping and contorting. I was mentally aware during the entire episode. I was also helpless. I could not control my own body. I didn't know when or if it would stop, only that I could not make it stop. Relief came when I was at last rendered unconscious, ending my suffering.

A great peace followed. I've often wondered, *Is this what death will be like?* All our suffering (or perhaps our sin) on earth strikes us all at once in the final seconds; and then in the presence of God, we achieve this ultimate feeling of peace, entirely void of fear, filled with love and understanding, the likes of which we have never experienced hitherto.

Well—spoiler alert—I did not die. I awoke on the floor (approximately some forty minutes later) conscious, in control of my body yet consumed with fear.

In retrospect I believe in the many months that followed, I indeed suffered from serious mental/medical anxiety. I have since been using anxiety medications, and I continue to pray and meditate (which is a strong part of my prayer life) about it.

I am still trying to overcome this newfound anxiety. I did see a neurologist about the seizure. I've been on a higher dose of anti-seizure meds ever since, and thus far, no more full-on seizures. Praise be to God. I do experience minor focal seizures from time to time, but they are manageable compared to the grand mal seizures.

Of course, anyone who has had brain surgery is at a higher risk of suffering a seizure, but I was three years out of surgery nearly when I had my first, which I'm led to believe is quite rare.

When dealing with the naturally heightened state of anxiety we feel as cancer patients, there are some natural remedies we can employ to help ease this suffering: prayer, meditation, Reiki, yoga, basic exercise, and counseling are all tools I have personally wielded and gained from.

To expand on any of these would take an entire book for each tool in its own respect. Ask your cancer family about any of these you are interested in. As a cancer patient, you should constantly be working on your physical and mental state of health. Optimizing these could have a significant impact upon your ultimate life span.

Stop: A couple of weeks after writing this, I was headed north in my truck to go fishing with my brother-in-law. All of a sudden that devastating rush overtook me; and I immediately pulled off to the side of the road, put the truck in park, and turned the emergency flashers on.

I remember looking to my brother and saying, "Alex, I'm going to have a seizure." Then I leaned back and waited in fear for it to come, trying to breathe like I had learned through meditation. In my mind I continued to repeat *Lord, save me. Lord, save me* over and over again.

Fortunately, Alex is a nurse, and he had his med bag with him. He remained so calm and reassured me, "If it happens, it happens. I'll be right here with you, bud."

I could not have had a better companion with me at the time. I did not have a seizure, but my blood pressure was 280/170. That's high enough to cause stroke.

I was able to get out after a few minutes and walk around the truck and climb in the passenger seat. I told him I still wanted to go fishing (he was on vacation, and I didn't want to ruin it for him), but he just smiled and said, "No, we can go fishing anytime." Thank God for his understanding because before we even made it to the nearest ER, the entire left side of my body was numb and I was cradling my left arm with my right arm.

I guess God wanted me to tell you it is okay to be on antianxiety meds, because several days later I was given some. Turns out I really had been suffering from medical anxiety for months since the seizure. I'm still stubborn I guess. I didn't want to admit it. Somehow, not being able to control my emotions made me feel emasculated. Friends, that is ridiculous. Do not be afraid to seek help or to take medications to treat your anxiety. I can't believe what a difference it has made. As cancer patients we have suffered great traumas, and those experiences can render anxiety upon anyone. I don't care how tough you are.

I had physical problems on top of the anxiety as well. I was put on a much stronger blood pressure medication to keep the levels down. I'm shortening all this of course. It took days and several doctor appointments to get this all taken care of.

Thanks to the new regimen of meds, I'm beginning to feel like myself again. I've been afraid to go anywhere or do anything for so long, and now that fear is finally receding. Remember God does not want us to live in fear. Do whatever you must to get rid of the fear so you can live out God's purpose.

Anxiety is something you should take seriously, which is why I spent an entire chapter focusing on it. If you are struggling with it, here are some excerpts from the Bible you can read and use in prayer:

Trust in the Lord with all your heart and do not lean on your own understanding. (Proverbs 3:5)

Cast all your anxiety on Him because He cares for you. (Peter 5:7)

That is why, for Christ's sake, I delight in weaknesses, in insults, in hardships, in persecutions, in difficulties. For when I am weak, then I am strong. (2 Corinthians 12:10)

Have I not commanded you? Be strong and courageous. Do not be afraid, do not be discouraged, for the Lord your God will be with you wherever you go. (Joshua 1:9)

That last one helped me get back out into the world. The Lord wants us to turn to Him, to rely on Him, so that when we are weak He might make us strong. God did not create us to be fearful, and if we put our trust in Him, we can come to know His love and peace.

Do not mistake your anxiety or your worries for a lack of faith. You are always going to have worries and concerns; these are meant to turn you to the Lord. He knew what He was doing when He made us. Although He made us capable of moving on our own, He did not assemble us with a built-in GPS. We still have to call on Him and ask for directions.

I believe that standing in the presence of God we will be completely devoid of fear for the first time and instead we will feel entirely consumed with love and understanding to the extent that we could never have deemed possible.

I look forward to feeling that.

CHAPTER 11

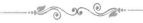

You Are Not a Burden

*See what kind of love the father has given to
us, that we should be called children of God; and so
we are. The reason why the world does not know us
is that it did not know him. (1 John 3:1)*

That includes you. You are a child of God. Therefore, your life
is just as sacred and meaningful as everyone else's. You tell me
that you are a sinner. Well, so am I. You tell me you are not worthy
of God's love. Neither am I. Yet I have God's love, and so do you.

*But God, being rich in mercy, because of the
great love which he loved us, even when we were
dead in our trespasses, made us alive together with
Christ—by grace you have been saved. (Ephesians
2:4–5)*

If you've been alive and living on earth for the past few years,
then you've probably heard of the movie *Deadpool*. The story's super-
hero is just a regular man in the beginning who soon gets diagnosed
with terminal cancer. He points out something that is so introspec-
tive about cancer it leads me to believe that either the writer must
have had some experience with cancer personally or this line was
divine intervention.

Regardless of the line's inspiration, the main character points out that the worst part about cancer isn't what it does to you but what it does to those around you. That is so true!

Aside from the added concern your loved ones now have about you, there are other burdens they probably bear now as well. For instance, I have to wear a device called Optune on my head most days. It is the biggest breakthrough in treatment for my extremely terminal type of cancer. Although it goes on my head, it is a pain in my butt.

The device forces me to rely on others because I cannot put it on myself. Trust me I have tried—tried and failed.

My life revolves around this device, and it is a major reason I remain isolated more than most. You see, the device has a cord coming out of the back that plugs into a machine, which resides in a small backpack that I have to lug around when I wear it. Sounds fun, right?

The Lord has truly taught me humility. For someone who was insistent on being his own tour guide, for someone who had to do everything his own way, now I am at the mercy of others, of their time and of their willingness to put the device on for me. It has to be changed every few days because my hair still grows and my head has to be shaved in order to wear the device as it sticks to your head (quite literally). It is not fun, but it's either that or my odds of the cancer returning increase greatly.

I am capable of growing a full head of hair. I was always proud about my hair as I have no natural balding. Now I am forced to be bald, but so what? I've gotten used to it.

The point is I felt like a giant burden. People have to stop what they are doing and put this stupid thing on for me like spoon-feeding a baby. I wrestled with it for a long time, and it even led to feelings of resentment when people could not or would not do it for me at times. At times I felt as though people were being snippy with me when I asked them to put it on, which made me stop asking for a while.

That was until one day I realized that if this were my son or brother or mother or friend who had to wear this thing, I would be happy to put it on for them and I would be empathetic. So why should I feel like a burden? I did not ask for glioblastoma, and although I get on my family's nerves from time to time, I'm pretty sure they do not wish to see me die. Pretty sure. Like 60 percent sure (haha).

The device still feels like it is a cross to bear at times, but I'm continuously adjusting to it. I've been tempted at times to throw it away and just live my life—grow my hair back and leave the house comfortably whenever I want for whatever I want.

But I don't. That would again be selfish. I need to stick around as long as I can for the sake of my children if no one or nothing else. So I have adjusted my way of life, and I live with it, but I am not a burden; I'm a child of God who has children of his own, and I'm leading them down the path to God (or at least showing them the path).

If you have cancer, you probably have to rely on people as well. You might need a driver to take you to your treatments, perhaps get you groceries, and pick up your prescriptions. Or maybe you're lucky enough to have this Optune device like me (yay, right?).

Either way, you are not a burden! If you don't have a good support group, find them. There are people willing to help. There are people who *want* to help you.

I know of a girl who gets rides and various means of help from other cancer patients. She doesn't have a lot of family around, but she has a cancer family. Don't be shy about seeking help. Did you ask for this disease? Probably not, right? To emphasize one more time, you are *not* a burden. You are a child of God with purpose.

CHAPTER 12

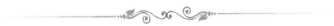

The Third Supremacy

There are three major supremacies of life. We have already hit on them a bit, but now we will focus on one in particular.

There is love, there is faith, and there is hope. Let us now talk about hope and how important it is.

When you have hope in your life, that's like walking down the boardwalk on a sunny day. The trees are green, the wind is a soothing breeze, and the birds seem to hum a song to your tune as you dance down the boardwalk by the seaside.

When you feel as though all hope is gone, that's like walking down that same boardwalk in the pouring rain. The waves crash upon the shore and spray you on the boardwalk, the wind is threatening to knock you down, and you are freezing cold and wet. The only birds around are the silent vultures that seem to be curiously awaiting your demise so that they might feast.

The weather's not always great, and we all are going to suffer, right? Yes, but as long as we have hope, hope that things can get better, hope that the sun can shine again, we can get through the roughest of times. That hope is God. He gives us hope because He loves us. We put our faith in Him, and in turn He gives us hope. My friends, we need hope. We need God.

I recently stumbled upon an acronym that read hope on a pastor's YouTube video that I just love. HOPE—Hold On Pain Ends.

When you have hope, you know that eventually your pain will subside, and everything will be all right. Sometimes all it takes is that sliver of hope that everything could work out for you to keep marching forward. As Christians we are blessed with hope, understanding that it comes from God. Even if things don't go the way we want them to go—and, yes, *even in death*—there is hope. We are all scared on some level to die. This is very human. I am scared to die, mostly due to the thoughts of my children and what that would mean for them. But beyond that, of course I don't want to die. Not yet. Why not? If heaven is so great, why be afraid to die?

I'm afraid to die because I still have hope, hope that things can still get better for me here on earth, hope that I may yet accomplish some of the Lord's work and overcome a few more obstacles, hope that I'll get to see my sons grow up, and even hope that I might meet my grandchildren someday. I hope the Lord grants me time to bring His plan for me to fruition. There are still people here whom I love, and I want to stay here and walk them down the narrow path to heaven's gate.

It has been said that a person can live for forty days without food, about three days without water, about eight minutes without air, but only a second without hope.

I have failed so many times in my life that it could be its own book: *The Dreams and Failures of One Joshua Sisco.*

I have never achieved what I set out to accomplish. This again refers back to my "self-tour-guiding days." I could sit back and reflect on all these failures until I have hollowed out and withered away, but I choose not to. I have God, and so I still have hope. Hope, by the way, was something I was starting to lose before even getting cancer. I learned a major life lesson from this.

Listen to what the famed Fr. Larry Richards has to say on this subject. "The devil will always keep you focused on yourself and your past. Jesus always calls you to look to Him and to the future."

The more and more you look to Him, the more you will feel hope, hope for your health and hope for a better future. You already have God's love, but you have *to love Him* in order to grow in faith, and only through that acquired faith will He then grant you hope; or as I like to call it, only then will you receive *God's grace*.

It is my astute belief that hope is crucial for us cancer warriors to not only obtain but retain throughout our battles and actually throughout our lives.

The following chapter is my physical and spiritual story with my personal encounter with cancer. I will also give you some sources where you can read inspirational stories from others. It is my intention that these stories will invigorate your hope.

When I was first diagnosed, I was told that the average expectancy for my life was around eighteen months. This was just over four years ago.

I began to read about it and to personally hear from others who were far exceeding their life expectations, winning their battles, and it gave me hope. There's something about watching other humans overcome this disease that blows open the door to that possibility in our minds.

I'll never forget the day I told my priest (now the infamous "water gun" priest) that the doctors had given me around eighteen months to live. He waved his hand dismissively and scoffed without a lapse in time as he retorted, "Ahhh, what do they know anyways?"

I'm not sure Father Tim realizes how much comfort those words gave and still give me. He was, of course, reminding me of the fact that only God knows when our time is up.

PART 3

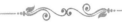

Harnessing Hope through Others

CHAPTER 13

My Story

I 've been hinting for twelve chapters that I would get to my story. This is what physically happened to me:

I was really busy ignoring all the signs that my health was deteriorating, working on a career in advertising while simultaneously attempting to achieve a master's degree in business (MBA).

I went to the gym at five thirty every morning, Monday through Friday. I was lifting heavier weights than I had ever lifted before in my life. People noticed when I took my shirt off, and I would get compliments. I was the healthiest I'd ever been in my life; or so I thought.

One day while doing pull-ups at my gym next to this incredible girl (Amber, I think) who could easily do just as many pull-ups as me, if not more, I suddenly felt an excruciating pain rush throughout my entire head. The pain was so severe I had to let go and drop from the pull-up bar. I remember her asking me what was wrong, and I recall answering that I wasn't sure but that I had a terrible headache. "Probably dehydrated," she suggested.

I remember standing on my porch in the morning and my ex-wife telling me I was spilling my coffee. I would hold the cup in my left hand, and I didn't even realize it was spilling until she said something. Still, I thought nothing of it. I told my mom about it (who is a neurotrauma nurse), and she agreed that I'd probably pinched a nerve lifting weights—not unthinkable by any means.

Then one day I was coaching my son's little league baseball team, and I found myself in the dugout, my head in so much pain that the other coaches had to take over the practice.

These headaches were really bad for about three days, and my left hand had become so weak that I actually dropped a coffee cup and shattered it on our porch.

On the third day of these "killer" migraines (no joke) was the morning my wife told me my face was drooping.

Then came the ride to the hospital. I was hemorrhaging in my brain when I got to the hospital. The next few hours leading up to an emergency craniotomy were fuzzy.

Fast-forward to when I was in the hospital. In terms of distance, I lived about two hours away from most of my friends and family at that time. But I was amazed at the number of people who came to visit me and all the support I received. It was the only thing that kept me going. It was love.

My parents of course, my siblings and their families, cousins, uncles, aunts, and so on were there. Later on I would discover that while in surgery, I had friends in Rome at a wedding praying for me. I had friends in Australia praying for me. My mother was posting updates on Facebook (unbeknownst to me), so everyone knew.

That love, those prayers, carried me through a six-hour brain surgery to remove a cancerous tumor, the deadliest form of brain cancer there is, stage 4 glioblastoma.

It is unbelievable that the tumor could have gotten that bad and my life had been so busy that it had virtually gone unnoticed, except for the headaches those last few days, which I had written off as migraines, and the weird "pinched nerve" I thought I had suffered from weightlifting.

I should've died. I've been told that so many times I can feel it. I know how close I was to crossing over. And I wasn't ready. I would have been lucky to make it to purgatory. Yet, in the midst of the flurry of somewhat conscious moments leading up to the surgery, I maintained an awareness that I might be dying. I told God that I would not leave my body because of my sons. Imagine that. I told God! I can assure you that God doesn't answer to me. I believe my intentions were so pure in that moment with the love for my sons that God listened. When I woke up in the hospital surrounded by friends, I shared that experience with them. I'm not sure why my wife was not a part of the reason for me wanting to stay alive (which she was quick to point out). In retrospect, I can only assimilate a premonition perhaps of what was to come.

Five days later I was up and walking out of that hospital and headed home toward a nauseating journey of recovery.

It's hard to explain to people who have never experienced such a traumatic event, but in the weeks/months to follow, it is almost as though you live on a different plane of existence, somewhere between heaven and earth. Maybe you've heard someone who survived a near-death experience speak of a "veil being lifted from their face" for the first time, and that is very accurate. You see the world much differently, much clearer.

I could see the world in a way for the first time that was so incredible that it is extremely difficult for me to put into words. The biggest thing I learned was that all the things I had been living my life for were extremely superficial and subsequently carried no importance or relevance at all. They didn't matter. Money, success, vanity—it's all meaningless.

It was G. K. Chesterton who said, "Meaningless does not come from the weariness of pain. Meaningless comes from the weariness of pleasure."

You've heard stories about extremely wealthy people on their deathbeds talking about how they wished they would have spent more time with family, especially kids if they had them. It's so true, again and again. Some people who commit suicide are not poor, quite the opposite actually. Yet we still glamorize that which would seek to destroy us. Why? It is the devil's trap.

We hear these things, and we nod and say silently to ourselves, "Yep, they are right." That realization somehow becomes utterly dismissed; and we go on worrying about the next big promotion, when we will be able to get a newer vehicle, how we can get more, and more.

It's all a bunch of cow dung. I didn't care about any of that in the months that followed my surgery. I didn't care that my career was over. Life as I had known it was over. I just cared about my kids and all the people who had been so kind and generous toward me in a terrible time of suffering.

After the surgery, the song "You Can't Always Get What You Want" from the Rolling Stones was stuck in my head. Rather, just the chorus was stuck in my head. For months I would listen to it every morning while I had coffee during my recovery. I found it liberating, and something about it gave me an energy every morning. I honestly don't recall listening to that song very often before my surgery. I'm sure I had heard it on the radio once or twice, but I had never *really listened* to it. At this trivial junction in my life, I found it to be so enlightening! All those things I had desired my entire life—the material things, the title of success, the feeling of superiority—I was never going to have, and for the first time in my life I was completely okay with it. I was just happy to be alive and grateful to all those who were there for me.

In the days following the surgery, I was stricken with a crystal-clear recollection of a line my priest had used once during a homily: "Life is about other people. If you aren't using your life to make other people's lives better, then, my friends, you aren't living right."

I would later tell him about that in a confessional booth, and he would smile and tell me he didn't remember saying it but that it sounded right. Well, Father, I heard it. And now I am listening to it.

I still miss my old priest and my old church parish, but I have found a new church and a new home where I'm at today.

I am fulfilling my passion by writing books. I don't drive a hundred-thousand-dollar car, and I never did get that mansion I always wanted. But I did get something better than all that: divine perspective. I get to be a good person. Priceless. Not a lot of those left.

My Spiritual Story

Unfortunately, that feeling doesn't last forever. The healthier we become and the more we begin to feel like "ourselves," the more we start acting like our old selves. It truly is a constant struggle for me to remember that feeling of grace that God had given me and the wisdom I achieved when that veil was removed. I crave that feeling though. It was the greatest gift He ever gave me. I realize how important it is for me to pray for that feeling and to stay close to God so that I may never forget it.

I can honestly tell you there is a difference between believing in God and knowing that God exists. It is better to simply have faith and to believe. It is hard to know. That can be confusing, I get it. It is kind of like this: If I believe in Santa and the spirit of Christmas, I'm excited to get up and see all that he has done for me in the morning. If I *know* he exists, however, while I may still seem excited, I'm also a bit nervous about the idea of him actually roaming around in my house in the middle of the night.

Given my experience, I can understand why God doesn't just make Himself known by showing up in the sky like every alien spaceship in every alien movie ever when they "make contact" right before destroying us. God is not an alien to us. After all, He made us in His image.

When we finally know that God exists, 100 percent and without equivocation, we will be standing in His presence. Then and only then will we truly be ready to know.

For everything our culture tries to shove on us in regard to how we should live our lives, the church has always taught us what life is all about. It's really simple. God made us to get to know Him, to love Him, and to serve Him in this world so that we might be happy with Him forever in the next (teaching from the catechism).

He also made us so that we may help those around us in times of need and be a light that shines upon the world, making it a little brighter for those around us. I once tried to explain this to my cousin, whom I love very much. She was not happy with this answer and actually seemed a bit flustered by it. "Is that it then? That's it?" was all she could really say.

I was frozen in the moment by her response. It's true. To be here for God and others is not very self-serving, is it? What about me? What about my life? It goes directly against the narrative of relativism and Western culture.

CHAPTER 14

Waking Up

I remember walking up to the church one day, as I couldn't yet drive, but my church wasn't far from home. We had gone to it only a few times, but I now understood how important it was for me to be there as much as I could be.

God had heard my plea about my children, and so I knew I owed him their lives as well as my own. I was able to get them enrolled in the catechism and made sure they went every Sunday when it started up in the fall. Both boys had already been baptized, but that was as far as they had made it into the church's sacraments.

Around this time blessings began raining down upon me. It was unlike anything I had ever experienced. People were very gracious with giving us money, which we greatly needed to be sure. I have an uncle who would stuff hundred-dollar bills in my pockets when I saw him. When I told him once, "You don't need to do that," he replied, "Well, it can't be very easy for you right now." He was right. It wasn't. I couldn't work.

Once, after the donations had all pretty much ceased, I found myself three hundred dollars short for the medicine I needed, and I couldn't dare ask anyone for it as everyone had been so gracious already.

Then I received a phone call one day from the park where I had my father's boat docked in a well. They told me about a street fair they had entered and had run a fundraiser. They had heard about my story and decided they wanted to donate the money to me. It was just over three hundred dollars.

God began to bless me like this consistently, and every night some family would bring us a hot meal and leave it by the front door. We didn't have to worry about cooking or groceries very much.

Eventually these little financial surprises ceased, but this went on for months!

In retrospect, God was trying to show me that everything I had been living for was so wrong, and I knew it was true. Also, I think He wanted me to know that He would provide for anything I needed. He still does.

I will share with you this final story of mine, the most amazing spiritual encounter I've ever had. Whether you choose to believe it or not is up to you, but I hope you do, and I know I'm not the only one to ever have an encounter of this magnitude.

I was falling deeper and deeper into my faith, and I'd recently read about this thing called adoration. It is where you sit in silence in a chapel before the physical presence of Jesus Christ in the Eucharist (if you do not believe in this, I kindly direct you to read *The Fourth Cup* by Scott Hahn).

My church didn't have a chapel, but a church close by did. The distance was too far to walk, but I really wanted to try adoration. Anything I could do to feel as close to God as I had in that hospital room I would try.

I spent the next couple of weeks researching it, even searching the internet for different ways to do adoration: What do I say? What do I do? For how long?

The church with the chapel held adoration on Tuesdays at a specific time. I must have looked at their website twenty times that week, constantly reminding my mother of when she had to drive me there, what day and time. I did not want to miss it! I was both diligent and precise about setting it up.

The day had finally come, and I was filled with excitement when I climbed into my mother's car. It was maybe a fifteen-minute drive before she dropped me off at the church. I thanked her and asked her to pick me up in an hour.

I walked into the building. After a bit of exploring, I found a sign that read "Chapel" and after a few more steps discovered the door. It was locked. How could this be? I checked the time on my phone. It should be open! Frantically I searched for an explanation, a posting with dates and times perhaps. This couldn't be happening. I'd planned it all so carefully. I found nothing.

With my head hanging and my heart heavy, I headed back out toward the front doors ready to call my mother. But then I saw a couple over my shoulder enter a door leading into the actual church where the pews and the altar were.

Curiosity clutched me by the shoulder, and a hope ignited inside of me as I turned and headed into the church myself.

The couple appeared to be kneeling on the steps in front of the altar. Out of respect I chose to sit a few rows back in the pew. The only lighting coming into the dim church was through the windows.

The couple was gone before I knew it, and there I was, alone in God's house. I poured my heart out to God that day. I'm not much of a crier, but the tears flowed freely. And then, Jesus Christ had a conversation with me. It is the realest thing I've ever experienced. It was more real than talking with a friend at a table in a coffee shop.

It lasted a long time, close to an hour; and then I just sat there in a state of total bliss, grace, and contentment, full of love and pure joy. Suddenly I noticed a woman sweeping between the pews, coming closer and closer to me. Remember it was still fairly dark inside, and here was this woman sweeping.

"You know the church isn't open, right?" the soft voice spoke to me.

I immediately began explaining to her that I was here for adoration but that for some reason the chapel was closed.

"The adoration chapel is open on Thursdays," she politely informed me.

"No," I cried out, "I looked at the website. It's always open on Tuesdays from such a time to such a time."

She smiled at me and assured me once again, "It's always Thursdays."

I apologized, thanked her, and headed out the front doors of the church just as my mother was pulling into the parking lot. I pulled out my phone and went directly to the website to prove that woman wrong, and I was dumbfounded to read adoration on Thursdays. I had checked it dozens of times. I had been so diligent! How could I have gotten it wrong?

I've since drawn this conclusion. God had scheduled the appointment with me on His time. The contents of what I learned there will forever be between me and the Lord. I will only say that it was not some worldly or heavenly wisdom that I gained; it was very personal. It is important, I feel, to simply share with you *that* it happened and nothing more. And so, for the first time since childhood, I was both physically and spiritually awake. Thanks be to God.

CHAPTER 15

Be Inspired

The best stories are the ones that come from people you meet in real life. As I said in chapter 2, find your cancer family. Meet people and hear their stories. Share your own. It is so therapeutic for you; and you will meet people who inspire you to stay strong, fight a little harder, and love a little deeper.

Aside from personal relationships, I did some research and found multiple sources filled with inspiring cancer stories of survivors. There are many YouTube talks about God and cancer as well that are inspiring. You need only to peruse the app to find them.

My book recommendation full of inspiring Christian cancer survivor stories is as follows: *Trusting God through Cancer: A Collection of Cancer Survivor Stories of Faith and Hope* written by Ed Adams. You can find it digitally or order it in paperback on Amazon.com.

There are too many blogs out there to mention, but one of my favorite sites is www.endurance.org. Not only does the site provide a blog with stories of hope but also has resources for things like counseling and support groups, and you can send prayer requests. If you believe in the power of prayer, put yourself on some lists. You are worthy of others' prayers, my brothers and sisters. I hope this book has inspired you in some way to turn to the Lord and put yourself in His loving arms. I would like to end by giving you this prayer to pray. I found this prayer on connectusfund.org and altered it slightly:

> Almighty God, when Your people cried to You in their trouble, You saved them from their distress (Psalm 107:19–20); so I cry out to You right now so that I may be saved from the distress of my diagnosis. Instead, I receive the Word that You sent out so that I can be healed (emotionally, spiritually, and physically) from this trauma and delivered from my destruction. I rely on the doctors to an extent (that the Holy Spirit may work through them for me).
>
> Ultimately it is in Your hands that I place my trust, my hope, and my faith. Amen.

If this book made a positive impact on your journey, please refer it to others. May God bless you.

ABOUT THE AUTHOR

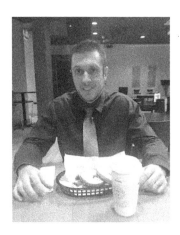

Joshua Sisco is a brain cancer warrior who currently lives in the small town of Hope, Michigan, with his two sons, Austin and Ashton Sisco. He is a devout Catholic Christian who considers his faith to be the cornerstone of his battle against cancer.

Joshua has worked in beverage factories and warehouses over the years. He has attended two universities and holds a single bachelor's degree. He worked in the field of advertising as a copywriter after college before his cancer diagnosis.

Beyond his faith, Joshua's interests are mainly outdoors and involve camping, fishing, hunting, snowmobiling, and making maple syrup with his extended family.

He also loves to travel, but due to his health and all that entails, he has been somewhat limited in his travels thus far.

Joshua continues his fight to stay alive so that he may fully raise his sons before going off to live with the Lord for eternity.

CPSIA information can be obtained
at www.ICGtesting.com
Printed in the USA
BVHW041214191222
654535BV00007B/374

9 781685 172930